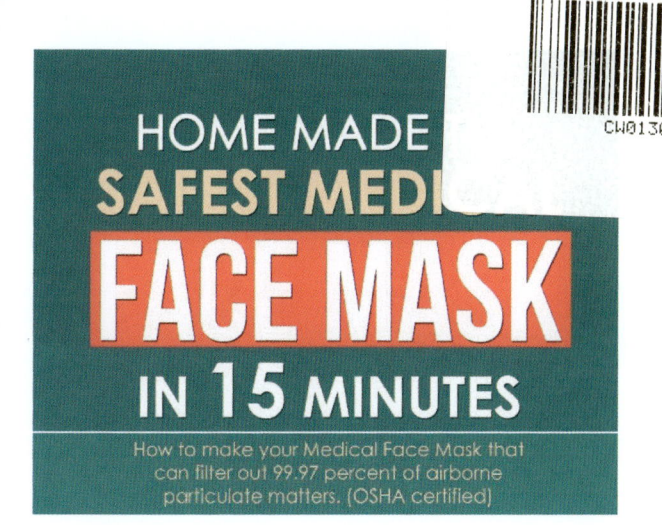

Copyright © 2020 Jinni Kardashian

All rights reserved.

ISBN: 9798636113805

Cover design: Laura

TABLE OF CONTENTS

Medical Face Mask History 5

Technical Indicators of Respirators and Medical Masks 8

Types of facial Mask 12

    A. Home-Made Face Masks 12

        Benefit from Handmade Facial Masks 13

        Risks of Homemade Facial Masks 14

        Can Homemade Masks Capture Smaller Virus Particles? 14

        Properties and Characteristics of Our Home-Made Medical Mask 15

    B. Surgical Masks 17

    C. Respirators 18

        Medical Protective Masks (AKA N95, KN95 Masks) 18

        Medical-Surgical Respirators Masks 23

How To Wear And Remove A Face Mask Correctly 27

    When Are You Supposed To Wear A Face Mask? 27

        How To Put On A Surgical Mask 28

        What Not To Do When Wearing A Surgical Mask 30

        How To Remove A Surgical Mask 30

        How To Put On A N95 Respirator? 31

    What Is The Safest Way To Manage Infection? 32

    Precautions for The Use Of Face Mask 33

    Can You Clean or Reuse Surgical Masks? 34

    Can You Reuse Face Masks N95 Or KN95? 35

        How to Disinfect N95, Or KN95 Face Masks 37

Step by Step On How To Make Our Home-Made Medical Face Mask 39

Why You Should Make Your Own Face Mask? 39
Step By Step Guide To Making Your Safest Home-Made Face Masks 41
    Homemade Facemask Pattern 47
Some Tips: When You Can Not Find Suitable Materials for The Mask 49
    Other Suggestions: Facemask Patterns 51

INTRODUCTION

If you work in the field of healthcare, you can understand and appreciate infection prevention and management. You would be delighted to hear that using disposable medical products is one of the safest ways to avoid infection.

You should be able to avoid an infection and be the cause of its spread. You have to understand that this is a very serious matter. Providers and patients must be conscious of the consequences of infection spread because the statistics are very disturbing and dangerous to prove.

Before the advent of covid-19 epidemic, the CDC (Center for Disease Control) estimates that 1.7 million people are infected with hospital-related infections, with about 1% dying annually, around 100,000 people dying due to hospital-related infections.

Now with coronavirus spreading extensively, this number is rather troubling, cause for change, and the use of disposable materials, in particular single-use disposable materials, is a way to minimize this amount.

When you are a health care provider, it is strongly recommended that you become a good example of protecting yourself and your patients by wearing these items. You should play your part in avoiding germ, bacteria and virus spread and defend yourself from fluid splatters.

Home-made mask made with safe materials can protect you and your family. You can make a face mask at home and also spice up your masks by choosing the most enjoyable, cartoon-type masks with their designs too but choosing the correct material is very important and attention must be paid to it.

You need to know which materials are suitable for face mask and how to make safest medical face mask easily at home with highly efficient filtering. This way you can decrease the risk of getting infected with covid-19 and breaking chains of this damned viral epidemic.

As a healthcare professional, besides material that should be used for efficient filtering and healthy to breathe, a wide selection of face masks can be chosen, whether ear-loops, anti-fogs, ties, cones, shapes or full-face masks types.

You can limit your options according to condition and circumstances in which you find yourself. With the difficult environment, some of these disposable items can only be expensive to use once, it is therefore necessary to ensure that you have a thorough analysis of the type you want.

You would definitely want to limit your type to the one approved by the Food and Drug Administration (FDA) and the Occupational Safety and Health Administration (OSHA), so that your masks are of high quality.

This GUIDE explores effective ways of making safest home-made medical face masks in 15 minutes alongside ways of wearing and maintenance for prevention of transmission of air-borne infections most especially Corona virus COVID-19.

By the end of this book, you will know how to make a face mask. What materials to use and why and even how by making these at home, you can help save lives.

Let's get started

CHAPTER 1

Medical Face Mask History

In 1895, a German pathologist study found a patient's wound infection was related to airborne infection. He claimed that sputum would carry bacteria and cause injury infection as people speak. Following his advice, doctors and nurses started putting on a gauze seam at that time.

A nose and mouth mask can reduce wound infection during surgery. Since that time, disposable facial masks have regularly been worn by medical personnel, food and sales staff and canteen cooks, particularly while food production and sales staff work.

Surgical personnel are expected to wear medical masks to protect patients from surgical wounds. Medical surgical masks are sufficient for the specific safety of the health care workers or associated personnel, as well as for safety against blood circulation, body fluids and spatter during invasive procedures.

Sustainable sanitation and workers in standby workplaces must also wear dust masks, which are also free for the relevant workers as labor insurance items. There are many people with anti-fog masks in the general population, especially during the season of the epidemics, who have played a positive part in preventing the spread of diseases.

From a medical standpoint, dust, bacteria, viruses and various harmful gasses are found in air which can enter through the nose, pharynx, trachea, which lungs through human breathing.

Wearing a disposable face mask ensures that the respiratory tract is "barred" in order to allow the inhaled air to absorb and avoid bacteria and viruses from entering the body. Around the same time, a mask can also protect the mouth and nose from wearing bacteria and viruses.

Wearing a disposable face mask can also reduce or prevent dust stimulation of the respiratory tract that can prevent or reduce occupational diseases.

Anti-virus masks should be used in workplaces with toxic and harmful particular odors to avoid occupational diseases triggered by inhalation of toxic and harmful gasses, such as benzene toxicity and organic solvent toxicity.

On average, 5% of hospitalized patients suffer from airborne-related infections, or 4,1 million patients in the European Union per year. Thirty-seven thousand deaths are caused by these infections per year.

Infective agents can be spread in many ways during procedures in operating theaters and other medical settings. The nose and mouths of the surgical team are one of the important sources. A person releases smaller or larger quantities of outlets of secretion from mouth and nose of the mucus while breathing, speaking, coughing or sneezing.

These droplets evaporate rapidly and leave airborne nuclei suspended. Nuclei will then travel to a vulnerable area through the air, such as an open surgical wound or a sterile device, or can be inhaled if the dimensions are very small.

The uses of Surgical Masks today go far beyond the medical and health care field in response to public concern. The epidemic of infectious diseases such as influenza has sparked a rising market for face masks. However, studies indicate that standard masks do not provide adequate protection since microbe-bearing particles can easily go through them.

Recently, surgical mask manufacturers have been working hard to create a face mask form called "respirator" Their security is much higher, since the stringent filter has a germicide that disinfects all products including microbes. They are used both domestically and globally in millions of medical departments, hospitals and clinics.

N99 Surgical respiratory machines with screening glue have a much higher antimicrobial protection than standard N95 masks that hold an elastic band in the nose.

The prevalence of airborne diseases and pathogens is no longer a mystery. Whether it is, H1N1 or avian flu virus or corona virus, the long-term survival plan involves first and foremost shielding people from respiratory infections.

There are concerns among health professionals that, when a microbe evolves, a highly infectious airborne infection will spread every day to the general public. Today, as in 1918, the devastating Spanish flu pandemic has killed an estimated 50 million people, this possibility remains.

Technical Indicators of Respirators and Medical Masks

Masks and respirators serve different purposes. it is important to grasp the distinction. Masks are usually worn loosely over the face, exploiting gaps between the mask and the face.

Masks ensures blockage of giant particles expelled by the user from reaching another person. They conjointly shield the sterile surgical field from contamination of exhaled particles.

Additionally, fluid resistant surgical masks facilitate scale back user exposure to blood and body fluids. N-95 respirators are designed to suit tightly to the face and build a seal between the face while the respirator are supposed to assist scale back the wearer's exposure to mobile particles and those generated by electro cautery, optical maser surgery and different power-driven medical instruments.

Breathers must meet the check requirements laid down in Code of Federal Regulations 42 CFR Section 84 in the United States. The student will review the legislation in order to fully understand all the test conditions.

The evaluation requirements for filter efficiency used by the US National Institute of Occupational Safety and Health (NIOSH) includes:

Sodium chloride test aerosol with a mass median aerodynamic diameter (MMAD) of around 0.3 μm;

A rate of air flow of 85 liters per minute (lpm); load neutralized test aerosol.

85 percent relative humidity (HR) and 38oC preconditions 24 hours before testing.

Typical surgical / process mask testing includes:

Efficiency in particle filtration (PFE)

Efficiency in bacterial filtration (BFE)

Fluid Resistance

Differential pressure and flammability

Each test is listed briefly below.

Particulate Filtration Efficiency (PFE)

The PFE test provides a standard measure for surgical / procedural masks in healthcare. The PFE check is not a breathing safety measure. However, when the NIOSH N95 testing method is used, the filter media of an operational / operative mask with a very high (> 95 percent) PFE can be less than 70 percent effective.

The results of the PFE and NIOSH filtration efficacy tests for the surgical / process mask should not be compared.

Conditions of test PFE include: aerosol polystyrene latex test; around 0.1 µm in size; 28 liters per minute (lpm) airflow rate; aerosol test not neutralized; and no pre-conditioning.

Bacterial filtration efficiency (BFE)

The American Society of Testing and Materials (ASTM) form F2101-01 is the research system used to determine BFE. This test tests the ability of a surgical / procedural mask to provide the wearer with a barrier to large particles.

It is not a replacement for a regulatory filtration check for the respirator and does not determine the ability of the operating mask to protect the wearer.

Fluid resistance

A fluid resistance test is typically performed using ASTM test Method F 1862, "Synthetic Blood Penetration Resistance" which determines the resistance of the mask to synthetic blood squeezed at different pressure.

Usually, the Delta-P test is conducted on the basis of "Method 1 Military Specifications: Operational Mask, Disposable (June 12, 1975)," MIL-M-36945C 4.4.1.1. Delta-P is the measured pressure drop on the surgical mask and is related to the breathing capability of the mask.

Differential pressure and flammability

Surgery / procedure masks for use in the operating room are checked with the goal of assessing the flammability by gender.

FDA allows the use of flammable materials in Class 1 and Class 2. The Food and Drug Administration of the United States (FDA) advises the use of one of the following criteria to assess inflammability.

Mask standards vary by region, each nation has its own level of approval for each form of mask. Europe for instance uses the standard EN 14683 for surgical masks, while China uses the standard YY 0469. -- Standard varies somewhat by country, but is largely similar.

With the urgent need for a mask, the world will become mask experts overnight. The job becomes much more challenging for these certifications. Here is a rundown.

Masks N95, N99, FFP1, FFP2 and FFP3.

Comparison of Respirators and Medical Masks

	FPP3 Respirator	Medical Mask
When to use	When carrying aerosol generating procedures (AGP) on a patient with possible or confirmed COVID-19 In high risk areas where AGPs are being conducted (e.g.: ICU)	In cohorted area (but no patient contact) Close patient contact (within one metre)
Use limitations	Subject to considerations of hygiene, damage, and increased breathing resistance Use may extend beyond 8 hours only if it is demonstrated that extended use will not degrade filter efficiency and total mass loading of filter is less than 200 mg	One-time use
Certification requirements	Certified by NIOSH under 42 CFR 84	FDA reviews 510(K) submission and clears for marketing
Filter elements	Nonreplaceable	Nonreplaceable
Filter efficiency	95%	Particle and bacterial filtration efficiency quality indicator
Testing aerosol and particle size	Sodium chloride test aerosol with a mass median aero- dynamic diameter particle of about 0.3 μm	Polystyrene latex sphere test aerosol approx. 0.1 μm and *Staph. aureus* filtration test, per ASTM standard (PFE)
Airflow rate	85 L/min	28 L/min
Test aerosol	Charge neutralized test aerosol	Unnaturalized test aerosol
Preconditioning	Preconditioning at 85% relative humidity and 38°C for 24 hrs	No preconditioning
Face seal fit	Designed to fit tightly to face Annual fit-test required	Not designed to fit to face
Fit check requirements	Required with each use	Not designed for fit check
Available sizes	Some models available in three sizes	Only one facepiece size generally available. Tends to produce more leakage on small facial sizes
Approximate cost	$0.70–$2.34 each	$0.28 each

Source: *National Personal Protective Technology Laboratory (2006)*.

CHAPTER 2

Types of facial Mask

What are the three main facial masks for COVID-19 prevention?

When you hear about face masks, there are usually three types:

- Homemade face mask
- Surgical masks
- N95 respirator

Let us discuss them in more detail below.

A. Home-Made Face Masks

The Centers for Disease Control and Prevention (CDC) has now recommended that everyone wear cloth-side masks like home-made masks, even in public places where it is difficult to keep 6 feet away from others, in order to prevent the spread of virus from individuals without symptoms. In addition to continuous social isolation and good hygiene procedures, this suggestion is highly recommended.

You should not place face masks on children under 2 years of age, people who have breathing problems, people who are asleep, or people who cannot remove the mask on their own.

Using 100% cotton cloth face masks instead of surgical masks or N95 respirators as such vital supplies have to be reserved for emergency workers and other first responders.

The DIY face mask movement which offers patterns and instructions for sewing masks at home tells you to use materials such as multi-layered cotton, elastic bands and common thread.

Overall, the designs involve basic folds with elastic straps to match your face. Some are more contoured to look like N95 masks. Others also have pockets to install "filter media" that you can purchase elsewhere.

Be mindful that there is no clear scientific proof that the masks are close enough to create a solid seal to conform to their face, or that the filter material inside works efficiently. For example, standard surgical masks are known to leave gaps. This is why the CDC stresses other steps, such as washing your hands and staying away from others.

They have not been developed to defend you against the acquisition of COVID-19. However, as other masks are not widely available, the CDC believes they can help slow the spread of coronavirus.

Benefit from Handmade Facial Masks

The facial masks can be made from ordinary materials at home and there is limitless provision.

This will reduce the risk of people transmitting the virus without symptoms by speaking, coughing or sneezing.

These are better than not using a mask and provide protection, particularly where isolation from society is difficult to maintain.

Risks of Homemade Facial Masks

They can offer a false sense of health. Although homemade facial masks provide some kind of protection, they are much less protective than surgical masks or respirators.

These will not eliminate or raising the need for additional protections. Proper hygiene and social isolation are still the best ways to remain healthy.

Can Homemade Masks Capture Smaller Virus Particles?

The scientists measured 0.02 microns Bacteriophage MS2 particles (5 times smaller than the coronavirus) in order to address this question.

The homemade caps, on average, produced 7% fewer virus particles than the big bacteria. All home-made fabrics, however, captured 50 per cent or more of the virus particles (except scarf 49 per cent). Only filter based homemade mask highlighted in this book can filtered out up to 99%. (see Properties and Characteristics of Our Home-Made Medical Mask)

Persons in infected area and sick people should be particularly be careful when using home-made facial masks. These masks should be used preferably in conjunction with a face shield which covers the whole face and side and extends to or below the chin.

NOTE: After every use, wash home-made cloth masks. Be careful not to cross your eyes, nose and mouth while removing. Wash hands upon removal immediately.

Properties and Characteristics of Our Home-Made Medical Mask

Coronaviruses may be transmitted by vapor (breathing) from person to person for up to 30 minutes and conversation, cough, sneezing, saliva and transmission over commonly touched objects.

In American medical settings, N95 masks should also be checked obligatorily by using a procedure developed before use by OSHA, the Occupational Safety and Health Administration. Home-made masks are unregulated, although some hospital websites suggest favored patterns. in CHAPTER 4 we report optimum pattern.

We will show you how to make a face mask. What materials to use and why and even how by making these at home, you can help save lives.

Many of you had started making homemade cotton masks in case our masks run out and we were out on the front line are very grateful for your support. However, hospitals, emergency rooms and medical staff are already on very short supply. And this virus has not even hit all our communities yet.

And, as nice as cotton is, it just is not designed to be a filter. The virus will still get through the small holes within the cloth. we believe that this is the best mask you can make it home and donate to your emergency medical services in your area. Why is that? It is mainly in the material. A standard HEPA filter. This is an ocean certified material that filters out 99.97% of airborne particulate matter per ocean standards.

We are confident that this mask will save lives. Now, as a physician, we have to give you a disclaimer, because this hasn't gone through rigorous testing, but I'm very impressed with the clinical results.

we wore this mask around the house for a prolonged period of time and even cooked bacon to see if I could clearly smell it. I could not. So, this looks to substantiate to me that each the fabric and also the seal work as supposed. It is also worth noting that any mask is better than no mask.

In fact, the CDC recommends in their current publication that, quote, I think that this specific material and design is the best that we can do at home in 15 minutes. Masks should seal to the face tightly to work.

The duckbill layout is especially common and with a stitching machine, some scissors and elastic with a regular HEPA filter you can achieve. Dr. R. Southworth, who is board certified emergency medicine physician and emergency medical services medical director certifies this method.

This is a safe face mask that if built properly should be donated to your local emergency services.

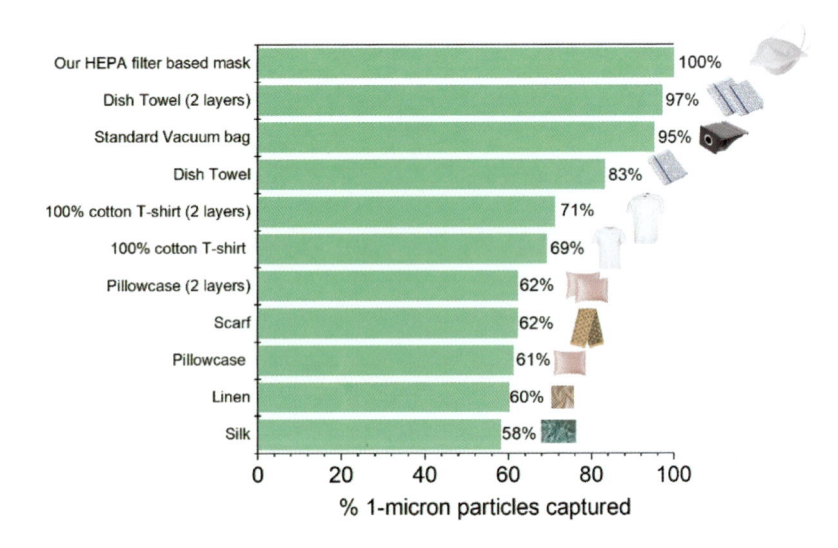

Material	% 1-micron particles captured
Our HEPA filter based mask	100%
Dish Towel (2 layers)	97%
Standard Vacuum bag	95%
Dish Towel	83%
100% cotton T-shirt (2 layers)	71%
100% cotton T-shirt	69%
Pillowcase (2 layers)	62%
Scarf	62%
Pillowcase	61%
Linen	60%
Silk	58%

B. Surgical Masks

The surgical masks are plastic face masks covering the mouth, nose and chin. They are loose-fitting.

A surgical mask is a loose fit, material that provides a physical barrier in the immediate environment between the wearer's mouth and nose. Surgical masks under 21 CFR 878.4040 are regulated.

Surgical masks should not be exchanged and may be classified as masks for surgery, isolation, dentistry or medical procedure. They can come with a face shield or without.

Surgical masks are manufactured in different thicknesses and are capable of shielding you from contact with liquids. Such properties can also affect how effectively the face mask can breathe and how well you protect the surgical mask.

While a surgical mask can cover large-scale droplets and splashes, a face mask, by its nature, does not filter or remove very small air particles that can be spread by coughs, sneezes or other medical procedures. Surgical masks do not always offer full protection from germs and other contaminants due to their loosened fit between the face mask surface and your skin.

Surgical masks should not be used more than once. When the mask is scratched or soiled, or if it becomes difficult to breathe through the mask, the face mask should be removed, securely discarded and replaced with a new mask. Place it in a plastic bag and drop it into the garbage to securely throw the mask away. Clean your hands after the mask has been disposed.

Usually they are used for: shielding the wearer against rubbing, splashes, and large particle droplets to avoid the transmission of potentially contagious respiratory secretions from the wearer to other surgical masks. The top of the mask has a metal strip to the nose.

Elastic bands or straight ties help to hold a surgical mask while you wear it. They can either be tied behind your head or looped behind your ears.

C. Respirators

A N95 respirator is a tighter face mask. This respirator can also flush out 95 per cent extremely small particles, in addition to splashes, sprays and great droplets, viruses and bacteria are also included.

The respirator is generally circular or oval in shape and is designed to shape your face tightly. Elastic bands help to hold it to your face firmly. Some types do have attachment known as exhalation valve that can contribute to heat and moisture buildup.

N95 respirators are not just one-size suits. In fact, they should be tested before use to ensure that a correct screen is formed. If the mask does not screen your face effectively, you will not be protected.

Users of the N95 respirators have to carry out a seal test every time they are worn. It is also necessary to remember that in certain classes a tight seal cannot be achieved especially when this involve children and individuals with facial hair.

Medical Protective Masks (AKA N95, KN95 Masks)

What is a N95 Respirator Mask?

Respiratory masks have received increased attention since late, although they have long been used for other purposes, including occupational health. N95 refers to the rating given to masks that meet the required minimum requirements for the transmission of particles by the National Institute for occupational safety and health (NIOSH).

The N95 respirator mask is designed for filtering up to 95% of airborne particles 0.3 microns or larger which may otherwise penetrate directly into the wearer's nose and mouth.

These masks can also be used by people with an infectious disease in order to prevent bacteria from entering the user's nose and mouth and endangering others. Although these masks do not protect against 100 percent particulate transmission, they do help prevent infection spread.

N95 masks can be bought without a valve to make breathing easier. The optimum protection is achieved if the respiratory mask snugly fits into the face and protects the nose and mouth without leaving empty spaces on the bottom. Air masks should be properly fitted to the wearer and should not be obstructed by facial or jewelry fur.

Respirator masks, used in industrial and health care facilities, are commonly used for occupational safety. The workplace masks used must be NIOSH-approved, meaning that they meet the minimum requirements defined by the National Institute for Safety and Health.

When purchasing respiratory masks, the intended purpose should be taken into account. Various types are designed for particular purposes and provide various levels of security. Another problem is that the mask contains latex, which is an irritation for others. There are latex free breathing masks N95 and they are labeled as such.

You may be in a position with a high risk of inhaling chemicals or fumes which are extremely harmful and dangerous to your health. You may be exposed to substances such as blood-borne or airborne pathogens that ensure that your employees are safe.

In fact, there is a law that tells you to protect your employees. Many companies claim to have healthy facial masks, but it is better to choose items that have the approval seal from the National Institute for Occupational Safety or the Administration of Food and Drugs.

These are your strongest assurance that your masks actually prevent you from contracting any pathogens in your vicinity.

You certainly want your workplace and your employees to be safe. It is best to ensure that your protection is assured when you are operating. The N95 mask is a very secure type of mask for your employees.

With great manufacturing efficiency, these masks will ensure the health of your workers. You do not need to have one type of mask, but you have a range of versions, as such masks are designed for various industries that may have special requirements.

When you heard of portable respiratory machines, they are no different from the N95 masks. You can filter and block soil, coal, iron ore, flour and dust. You can be confident that other related materials can also be blocked.

You can also be sure that diseases such as influenza and tuberculosis can be avoided if you correctly use these disposable respirators. For a disposable respirator, you would have the additional advantage in that you have a built-in respirator. It is more than a basic mask; you can be assured you have a good amount of oxygen.

You might be interested in those, but you need to be wary of the price tag. However, you do not have to worry too much because when you order a mask from a manufacturer in bulk, you will definitely hit your price goals. And all of these lightweight respirators and N95 masks are well within the price range to help you sleep better at night.

The N95 is the most common series of particulate breathing masks, which comply with US government standards. The face masks are tested to reduce exposure of NIOSH, the National Institute for Safety and Health, to airborne contaminants.

The letter shows how the filter is tested in oil aerosol environments:

N95, N99 and N100

N99 Respirators are usually latex-free in their looks and have a much tighter mesh that removes almost all airborne products. They often close holes across the nose and facial sides.

This adhesive does not allow air to be inhaled when the N99 grade filter passes. This is super quick to breathe and should be taken into account when planning for any pandemic.

These filters are not intended for use with oil aerosols. This should be used in conditions where particles do not contain oil are exposed. N- Respirators may also be reused many times.

R95, R99, and R100

These filters are immune to oil. In atmospheres containing debris, r-respirators may also use either liquid or solid hazards, including oil-based hazards. These are masks for one-time use.

P95, P99 and P100

These filters are oil resistant. Such breathers can be used in any area that is exposed to dangerous particles. The p- respirators are subject to time limits.

The filter efficiency number refers to the percentage of airborne particles extracted in the test:

22

95%, 99% and 100%

If a mask is NIOSH certified, a class approval stamp will be printed on the respirator.

Licensed NIOSH masks are also available in various sizes, and a well-suited mask is essential.

Before choosing the correct mask, it is also recommended that you make an evaluation of your particular environment with qualified industrial safety staff.

I am not the kind of person who is constantly concerned about germs in my life or washes my hands 50 times a day. Sure, after using the toilet or before meals, I will touch the soap and the wash, but other than that, I live the philosophy that a little dirt never hurts anyone.

In reality, you can expose your immune system to a variety of germs. Of course, it only works to a certain degree, and when I realize that I am going to be exposed to more germs than normal I take precautions. For starters, I am sure I have many disposable face masks with me when I fly or take other type of public transportation.

Most people know about two types of disposable facial masks.

The first kind is the thin paper or fabric worn by surgeons. Then there are disposable face masks designed for more extreme uses on construction sites or if the carrier realizes that he / she has more harmful germs than those that transmit the common cold.

These disposable face masks are constructed of a variety of materials and shaped to tightly cover the mouth and nose. Often they have a breathing system on them and are designed to flush out more than 99% of the toxins in the air around them.

N95 disposable face masks are perhaps the most well recognized since the swine flu outbreak came out several years ago and clearly advised by health professionals. This is the kind of mask I fly with. I do not always wear it, but if someone coughs and hacks in my side for a long time, you would better believe that I would put the mask on.

I do not know what other people will think or the strange looks I am sure I will get. Staying alive is much more important to me than the views of other people.

Nevertheless, disposable face masks are not expensive, so there is no reason not to purchase one or two of them and transport them when you are flying or close to a few foreigners for a long period.

You never know what could happen and certainly better than sorry to be free. It is not an alarmist; it is realistic. As I said, I do not generally freak out germs, but sometimes are important for precautions.

Medical-Surgical Respirators Masks

There is a confounding selection of medical supplies on the market. Several of them can only be called for by a healthcare professional while others are recognizable to any layman such as bandages, gloves or surgical masks.

Such medical supplies are also used in regular daily life by ordinary people. For example, most people use their own first aid and bandages for shallow wounds. Often factory staff and those employed in spas and beauty rooms use surgical gloves. The same applies to the surgical mask.

The operation mask is often called a procedure mask and is available in shops that sell medical supplies, or even in your local pharmacy. This mask consists of three layers or a three-fold cloth with a molten substance between non-woven textiles. The melt-blown coating removes bacteria and microorganisms through the mask.

As the name suggests, the surgical mask was mainly intended for operations by surgeons and their teams.

Since surgery may be very ambiguous and involve being exposed to different forms of organic fluids, it is important to prevent blood and other substances splashing into the face of doctors and nurses as well as to cover clothing and hands with surgical robes and gloves. This is also why the masks are used in animal dissections to teach the concepts of anatomy by students.

Another reason to wear a surgical mask is to prevent disease transmission. These medical supplies are designed to provide bidirectional security. If the medical practitioner is exposed to infectious diseases such as grippe, the patient is prevented from passing on this disease.

It also protects patients from microorganisms or diseases, which a physician or nurse may otherwise unknowingly spread. In cases where a patient has a weak or suppressed immune system, this is extremely important.

The mask often prohibits doctors and nurses from rubbing their nose or mouth unconsciously, when their hands may have come into contact with polluted surfaces.

In societies such as Japan, a mask can be used as a kind of courtesy when a person suffers from a cold or another disease that can easily be passed on from one individual to another. It is therefore relatively normal to see somebody wearing a mask on a Japanese train or market.

To optimize usage and protection from medical supplies such as the surgical mask, they must be used in compliance with the specified directions. The holder will make sure to wash his hands before putting it on the mask.

The mask, normally consisting of three parts, should be worn over the nose with the metal band, and extended over the mouth and the chin. Ties go over the ears and under the ears around the neck. The mask should be properly discarded and not reused.

If you want to make sure you do not get airborne diseases, wear a surgical mask when you go to places overcrowded. This is particularly recommended for those with low immunity.

Wearing a mask is one way to reduce the risk of being infected with a flu virus. The effectiveness of the mask varies with several factors such as how you wear it, the type of mask you choose and the appropriate disposal techniques.

There are a few different types of masks. The first one is a soft, flexible mask which binds around the head. These are normally moderately priced and come in huge numbers. These are also called surgical masks.

A second, more costly type of mask is the shape-fitting kind that fits around the face comfortably for snug fit. These types consist of thin fibers which filter out particles that enter during respiration.

Surgical masks are designed to protect doctors from mucus and other fluids, which patients project into the air. They can remove 95% of most small particles and are successful against the flu virus.

To achieve better protection for flu viruses in a market mask, look for one with or higher N95 scores. The N95 mark is an FDA label that tells you how much protection you get.

It is necessary to put your mask on properly so it works. Put the mask over your face and snugly tie it up. There are no holes or gaps on the edges you like. Any failure can be a convenient way for germs to reach, because the air inhaled can bypass the filter entirely.

Wear the mask while approaching various scenarios. Maintain wearing the mask until you left the field. Removal of the mask may allow the virus to land within the material and cause the mask to breathe in. If you look after a person who is sick (maybe your child) you can protect yourself by wearing a mask.

Consider wearing a mask while you are ill in order to prevent anyone from contracting the illness. Whether you pick a surgical mask or some other kind, when you are around strangers, you will feel more relaxed. The flu virus can be frightful, but you can protect yourself and others by taking preventive steps.

Protection is not always straightforward, but there are several straightforward ways to defend against viruses and germs at any time of the year.

We also seek to find ways to defend ourselves from a flu outbreak. There are also stories about what works and what does not. The use of masks, often hand washing, hand cream or chemical sanitizers, are some of the protective steps we are all aware of.

While the only way to prevent this for all of us is to prevent busy environments and communal areas that can quickly transmit the flu virus. But then again, not all of us simply have the option of staying home and waiting for things. Learning, job and travel carry us all to the same location.

CHAPTER 3

How To Wear And Remove A Face Mask Correctly

Wearing a face mask also allows people to feel secure and comfortable. However, can an surgical face mask prevent you from being exposed to or transmitting such infectious diseases?

And, if face masks protect you from infectious diseases, such as COVID-19, is there any way of putting them on, removing them and discarding them?

Continue reading to find out.

When Are You Supposed To Wear A Face Mask?

The World Health Organization (WHO-Trust Source) recommends that you wear a mask only if you:

Have a fever, cough, or other respiratory symptoms, but look after someone with a disease of the breath. In this case, wear a mask if you are within 6 feet or nearer to the person who is ill.

This is because surgical masks: do not remove smaller particles from the air do not fit snugly on the face, so airborne particles can leaking in the mask's sides Some studies have been unable to prove that surgical masks effectively prevent exposure in group or public spaces to infectious diseases.

The Reliable Source Centers for Disease Control and Prevention (CDC) officially does not prescribe the use of surgical masks or N95 respirators to the general public in order to protect against respiratory diseases like COVID-19.

In the case of COVID-19, however, the CDC advises the public at large to wear cloth facial covers to prevent disease transmission.

In chapter 4 we report step by step how you can build a safest mask at home.

How To Put On A Surgical Mask

A surgical mask is a loose-fitting, rectangular shaped, disposable mask. The mask has elastic bands or straps that can be tied behind your eyes or looped behind your ears. The top of the mask can be modified with a metal strip to match the mask around the nose.

A correctly worn 3-ply surgical mask can prevent the transmission from droplet, spray, splatter and splash of large particle microorganisms. The mask can also reduce the chances of hand-to-hand contact.

The three-fold layers of the surgical mask function:

The outer layer repels water, blood and other body fluids.

Some pathogens are removed by the middle layer.

The inner layer removes sweat and moisture from exhaled air.

The surgical mask edges, however, do not form a tight seal around your mouth or nose. Therefore, minute airborne particles like coughing or sneezing cannot be flushed out.

If you need to wear a surgical mask, take the following steps to correctly wear it.

Steps to put on a facial mask

Wash your hands with soap and water for at least 20 seconds or rub your hands thoroughly with an alcohol-based hand sanitizer.

Check for facial mask defects like tears or broken loops.

Put the colored side of the mask to the outside.

When present, make sure that the metal strip is at the top of the mask and positioned against your nose bridge.

If the mask has the ear loops, then hold the mask with both loops and place a loop on each ear.

Ties: Keep the upper strings of the mask.

Tie the top strings in a secure bow below your head's crown.

Keep the lower strings tight in a bow close to your neck.

Dual elastic bands:

Pull over your head the top band and place it against your head's crown. Pull the bottom band over your head and set it against your back.

Place and pinch the bendable metallic upper strip into your nose form and press with your fingertips.

Bring the mouth and nose to the bottom of the mask.

Ensure sure that the mask suits perfectly.

When in place, do not touch the mask.

If the mask is soiled or wet, swap it with a new mask.

What Not To Do When Wearing A Surgical Mask

There are a variety of steps to be taken after the mask is properly worn to avoid the movement of pathogens onto the face or hands.

Do not:

Touch the mask until the mask is fixed on your face, as pathogens may move from the ear,

Hang the mask around your neck,

Reuse single-use masks if you have to touch the face mask while wearing it, first wash your hands. Make sure to wash your hands or use a hand sanitizer afterwards as well.

How To Remove A Surgical Mask

It is vital that the face mask is removed properly to ensure that no germs are passed to your hand or face. You do want to make sure that you securely remove the mask.

Steps to remove a mask

Wash your hands well or use a hand sanitizer before taking the mask off.

Stop touching the mask itself, because it could be dirty. Keep it only by loops, links or bands.

Remove the mask carefully from your face until you: first unhook the ear loops, unload the bottom loop or then remove the bottom band by raising it over the head and do the same with the top band Holding the mask loops, tie or strings.

Wash your hands thoroughly or use a hand sanitizer after removing the mask.

How To Put On A N95 Respirator?

N95 respirators are tailored to your face size and shape. Since they suit your face more snugly, airborne particles have less chance to spill around the mask's edges.

N95 can also more effectively filter small airborne particles

The trick to a successful N95 is to make sure it suits your face properly. Health professionals providing direct care are tested annually by a qualified professional to make sure their N95 fits well.

A correctly designed N95 respirator normally filters pathogens much better in the air than a surgical mask. Carefully checked and approved respirators for N95 classification will block up to 95 percent of tiny (0.3-micron) particles. Yet they have their limits as well.

Follow these simple steps when attempting to suit a N95 mask or other particulate respiratory mask:

1. Put the mask (respirator) tightly on your nose bridge against your face with your external nose piece.

2. Stretch and place the top headband over your ears on the back of your head. Stretch the headband over your head and place under your ears.

3. Mold the metal nosepiece to your nose with both hands.

4. Cup both hands over the breather and exhale vigorously for test suit. If air flows around the nose, close the mask: if air flows around the breathing edges, reposition the headbands to suit better and check again before air escapes.

The best way to prevent infection is, according to the FDA, to limit exposure to the virus. It advises social distancing and regular washing of hands.

The findings of a 2016 systematic review and meta-analysis showed no major difference in the use of N95 breathing masks by medical personnel for preventing the transmission of acute respiratory infections in clinical conditions.

These findings were supported in a recent randomized clinical trial published in the JAMA journal in 2019.

What Is The Safest Way To Manage Infection?

If you have a respiratory illness, avoiding others is the only way to prevent transmission. It is the same if you want to stop a virus.

In order to minimize or come into contact with the chance of transmitting the virus, the WHO suggests the following:

Practice good hygiene in the hands by periodically washing your hands with soap and water for at least 20 seconds.

If you do not have access to soap and water, use a hand sanitizer which contains at least 60 percent alcohol.

Do not touch your nose, your mouth and your eyes.

Maintain a safe distance from others. The CDC recommends a minimum of 6 feet.

Stop visiting public places until you fully recover.

Stay at home and relax.

The Surgical Masks can protect against larger particles in the air, whereas N95 respirators provide better protection against smaller particles.

Addressing and removing these facial masks correctly will help protect you and your wellbeing from transmitting or contracting pathogens.

Although facial masks may minimize the spread of certain disease-causing species, evidence suggests that using facial masks does not always prevent you or others from being exposed to such pathogens.

Precautions for The Use Of Face Mask

A standard mask or a surgical mask is intended to avoid large-scale droplets, sprinkling, spraying, or sprinkling that may involve germs (bacteria and viruses) from entering your mouth and nose.

The FDA adds:

"While a mask for surgical purposes may be effective in blocking larger particle droplets, the face mask, by its nature, does not remove or block very small particles that may be transmitted in the air through coughs, sneezes, or other medical procedures.

Surgical masks will also limit exposure of the saliva and other respiratory secretions. This is why people in the UAE are advised to wear masks in confined spaces with flu or cold symptoms.

WHO adds that masks can only be effective when used in combination with frequent hand cleansing, hand rub or soap and water based on alcohol. The manner in which you use the mask decides whether your mask is okay.

If you do want to wear a mask, it is important to do this:

-- Clean your hands before wearing a mask, wash them or use an alcohol-based hand sanitizer.

-- Cup your mouth and nose to make sure there are no holes between your face to mask.

-- Do not touch the mask while you use it. If you touch the mask, wash your hands or use a hand sanitizer based on alcohol.

-- Use the strings to cover the mask and do not touch the front of the mask. In the garbage, dump it.

-- Immediately wash your hands with water and soap or use a sanitizer based on alcohol.

-- Do not touch the mask front of your neck or pull it up your head.

-- Do not use the mask when it is wet.

Can You Clean or Reuse Surgical Masks?

I did not find a prescribed blue type surgical mask cleaning technique. These masks cannot be washed because they can damage the mask by washing them. However, surgical facial masks can in principle be effectively disinfected using UVGI as mentioned above strictly for a single use.

The CDC provides the following guidelines for restricted reuse:

If soiled, damaged or difficult to breathe, the facemask should be cleaned and discarded.

Not every facemask can be reused.

Masks that attach to the provider through bonds cannot be undone without tearing and should only be considered for extended use instead of reuse.

Elastic ear hook masks can be more fitting for reuse.

HCP will exit the patient's area of treatment if the face mask is to be removed. Facemasks should be plied carefully so that the outside surface is kept in and against the surface during storage to minimize contact with the outer surface. The folded mask can be placed in a clean sealable paper bag or breathable jar between uses.

Can You Reuse Face Masks N95 Or KN95?

If appropriate, N95 or KN95 face masks should always be replaced.

The CDC has guidelines for expanding and restricting the use of N95 masks in periods of minimal supply: to reduce the number of people who need to use respiratory security by selective application of engineering and administrative control; to use alternatives to the N95 respirator (for example, other filter classes of fake respirators, elastomeric semi mask and full facial mask).

If the use of facial masks is increased, the following steps should be taken to reduce contact transmission after wear:

Discard N95 respirators after use in aerosol generation procedures.

Discard N95 respirators from any patient co-infected with an infectious disease, upon close contact with or from the treatment area requiring contact precautions.

Try using a clear face shield (preferred 3) for the care of a N95 facemask and/or other measures to minimize surface contamination (e.g., masking patients, use of engineering control).

Perform hand hygiene with soap and water or a hand sanitizer with alcohol before and after touching or changing the respirator (if necessary for comfort or fitness).

In case of reuse of facial masks, the CDC recommends the following steps to minimize post-wear contact transmission: Discard N95 respirators after aerosol production.

Reject patients with N95 breathable contaminated with respiratory or nasal secretions or body fluids.

Discard N95 respirators after near contact with any infectious disease patient needing touch precautions.

Try using a sterile facial shield (preferred3) over a N95 respirator and/or other measures (for example, masking patients, engineering control) to reduce the contamination of the airframe on the surface.

Hang the air breathers in a designated storage area or keep them between uses, breathable container such as a paper bag.

Containers for storage should be periodically disposed of or washed.

Clean hands before and after handling or changing the respirator with soap and water or an alcohol-based hand sanitizer (if necessary for comfort and fitness).

Stop hitting the respirator inside. If the breathing system is affected unintentionally, discard the respirator and perform hand hygiene as mentioned above.

Use a pair of clean (non-sterile) gloves to apply a used N95 respirator and to conduct a seal inspection. Discard gloves after the N95 respirator has been mounted and all changes made to make sure the respirator sits comfortably with a good screen on your forehead.

Also, the same person can expand or reuse the masks, as asymptomatic wearers can probably spread infection.

How to Disinfect N95, Or KN95 Face Masks

The sterilization and cleaning of KN95 N95, and face masks is expected to increase as many of them now use this type of PPE.

Because of minimal supply, medical staff and ordinary citizens alike can have to use their facial masks again. This chapter sheds some light on various styles of face masks and on how they can be cleaned of viruses.

How to clean and clear masks of the face of fabric

The face masks of cloth should be regularly washed. The Public Health Department of California recommends every day or after every use.

Tissue masks should be washed using hot water detergent and dried during a hot cycle in order to kill the bacteria and microbes.

Basically, the secret is hot soapy water. Soap can break down the virus 'protein coat and is highly successful.

If you have to use your mask again before you can wash it, it is recommended that you wash your hands immediately after you put it back on to stop touching your face.

Here are some general cloth mask recommendations from the California Dept of Public Health:

Face coverings may be made of bandanas, scarves, t-shirts or towels, factory manufactured or hand-stitched or handmade.

The material will cover both the mouth and the nose.

Ideally, after each use, facial coverings should be washed. Dirty masks should be disposed in a designated laundry bag or bin.

When washing masks, use detergent and hot water and dry them on a hot cycle.

Be sure your mask is comfortable; you do not want to have to continue to change the mask, for that means to touch your nose.

Wash the hands before and after touching the facial or face coverings, or using the hand sanitizer.

When you need to wear the face of your cloth again before washing it, wash your hands thoroughly after you put it on and avoid touching the face.

Cloth masks do not completely shield the wearer from air viruses but can help to protect others by barricading the virus 'biological aerosols or "droplets."

CHAPTER 4

Step by Step On How To Make Our Home-Made Medical Face Mask

Why You Should Make Your Own Face Mask?

Many people are purchasing chirurgical masks to guard against this deadly disease of highly infectious coronavirus (COVID19) spreading rapidly across the world.

The sudden rise in the market for "personal protective equipment" (PPE) and the broken supply lines in China led to a critical shortage of small filtering particles face masks (N-95), and rectangular sneeze safety ("chirurgical masks") mounted.

Media reports, which were properly intended to reserve for medical institutions restricted supplies of such disposable products, told people not to purchase these things. Public officials have been quoted saying – inaccurately – that face covers cannot prevent this new virus from spreading.

The reality is more complicated: COVID19 spreads in outlets with water, mucus and saliva from individuals that have infections. These viral particles have been brought into the air through coughing, sneezing and even regular breathing. Thousands of droplets can be removed with a sneeze.

Individuals less than 6 feet away can be coated with these virus particles when in the air. The virus particles will remain active for up to nine days after the droplets break.

Infection takes place when someone breathes through airborne droplets, or when the hands with viral particles come down out of the air on opponents, hand bars, floors or other surfaces touch his mouth, nose or eyes.

Using a face mask prevents individuals from being tainted in two ways:

1) by removing most airborne virus-filled droplets.

2) by preventing the wearer from touching his or her own mouth and nose.

Researches indicate that the surgeon who correctly uses surgical facial masks experiences 80% fewer infections than those who do not.

Why the mixed messages, Then?

First, because the protection comes only if the masks are correctly used, it depends on which situation you are in, and also they should be cleaned and carefully removed without touching the face.

Furthermore, since the mask and fiber gaps are too large, even in trade surgical masks, to block all viruses. Surgical masks and certain tissue masks are going to block 7-micron particles. The virus particles of COVID19 are between 0.06 and 0.14 microns.

So why are you supposed to make your own face masks?

1) When you become sick, getting a supply of masks at home will give friends and family a degree of security as you seek medical advice. It would probably be better than no mask.

2) With the production of your own, and ideally for family and friends, you can reduce the need for the limited supply of imported industrial equipment that hospitals and nursing homes desperation.

3) These convenient, curved masks are more facially made, with less gaps than the rectangular surgical masks.

4) Our handmade prototypes are fitted with two fabric layers and with a filter in between them which can filter out of airborne particulate much, much better than a cotton mask.

Step By Step Guide To Making Your Safest Home-Made Face Masks

There is one thing you should learn before you immerse yourself in the debate about masks:

Homemade masks do not replace social isolation and staying at home. Do not use any material to make mask if you're not sure it is healthy to breathe in using it.

If you want to make a safest homemade mask, here are step by step directions – based on guidelines given by the board certified emergency medicine physician and emergency medical services medical director and Chris Holmes.

You can use this mask in any urgent situations that arise when you leave home.

Before you can sew your facial masks, ensure that no one in your home is currently showing any symptoms or has been diagnosed with Covid-19.

Before starting this project. Please wash your hands thoroughly with soap and water. Also, be sure to use the first mask you make as both a test of quality and to ensure that you do not breathe on any of the other masks you produce. Transport these in a clean and safe state.

First of all you need the following materials:

- ➢ Pipe Cleaners
- ➢ Elastic
- ➢ Hot glue gun & glue
- ➢ Thread
- ➢ Pencil
- ➢ Sewing machine
- ➢ Scissors
- ➢ Printout of mask template
- ➢ HEPA filters or MERV16 filters

You can use

- ✓ Healthy Climate air cleaner Filters
- ✓ Ultrafine CPAP Filters (you can fix them close with Hot glue gun on a fabric)
- ✓ HEPA vacuum Bags

NOTE: HEPA vacuum Bags Should be Quality Manufactured WITHOUT Fiberglass or Any Other Materials That Are Harmful to Breathing Passages and Respiratory Systems

Here are some links that you can find filter materials

Ultrafine CPAP Filters

Hoover Type Y HEPA Filter Bag

Kenmore 53292 Style Q HEPA Cloth Vacuum Bags

Lennox X8314 MERV 16 Expandable Filter

Lennox X5424 MERV 16 Filter

Lennox X5424 - PMAC-20C MERV 16 Replacement Filter

Directions

1. Cut 4 pieces of fabric using pattern below. (I used 2x cotton t shirt for exterior, 2x cotton/poly blend for inside.)

2. Cut 2 pieces filter material. I used Lennox X8314 MERV 16 Expandable Filter

3. Cut 2 x 10" elastic band

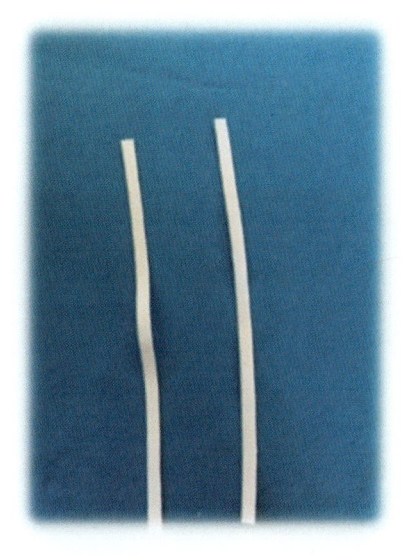

4. Take one pipe cleaner and bend it in half or Cut ¼" × 6" bendable metal (I used aluminum weather flashing, but 12-gauge copper wire, wired ribbon, aluminum takeout works.)

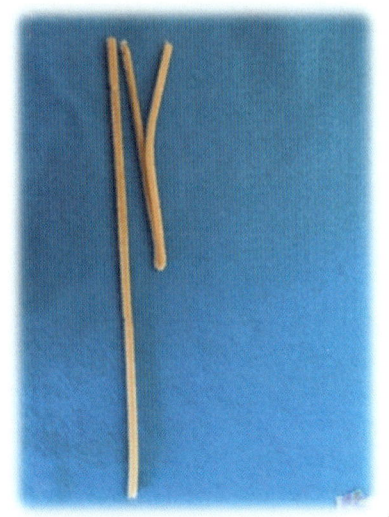

or

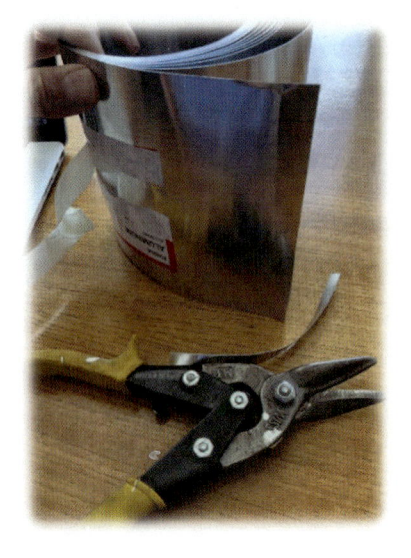

5. Sew along top of outer fabric, inner fabric, filter. (right side fabric facing each other).

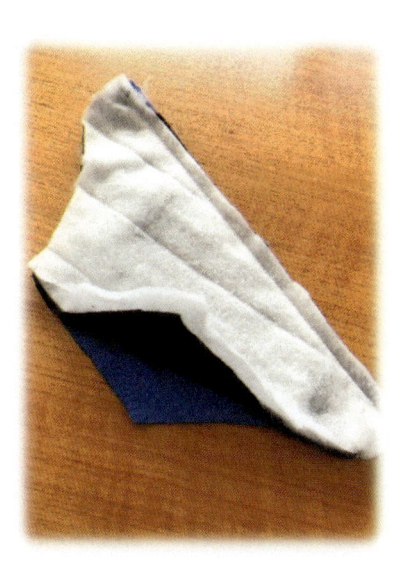

6. Flip right sides of fabric out. Center bendable metal or pipe cleaner along top put hot glue on one side of bendable metal. Let glue cool a little. If it is too hot it will melt the fabric. Once cooled a little, attach bendable metal to mask or you can also sew around the strip to keep it in place.

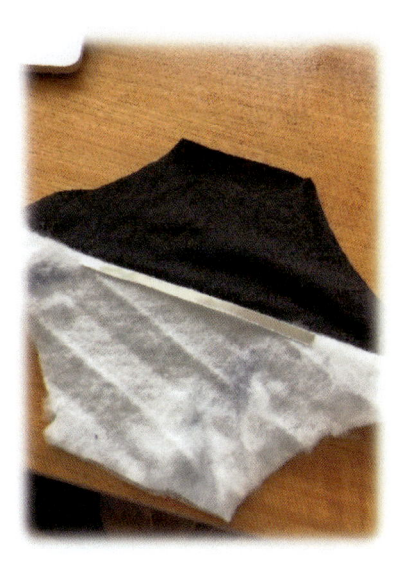

7. Place upper and lower portions of duckbill together outside fabric facing inward.

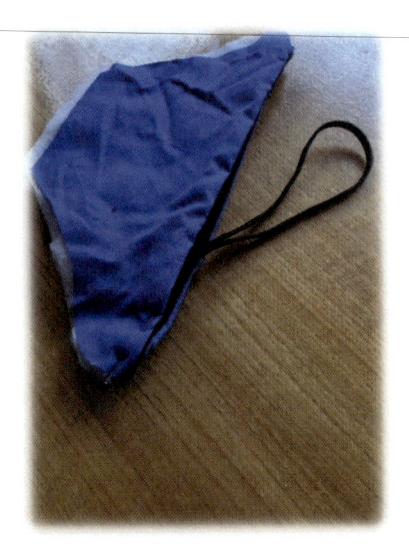

8. Place elastic near top as shown below.

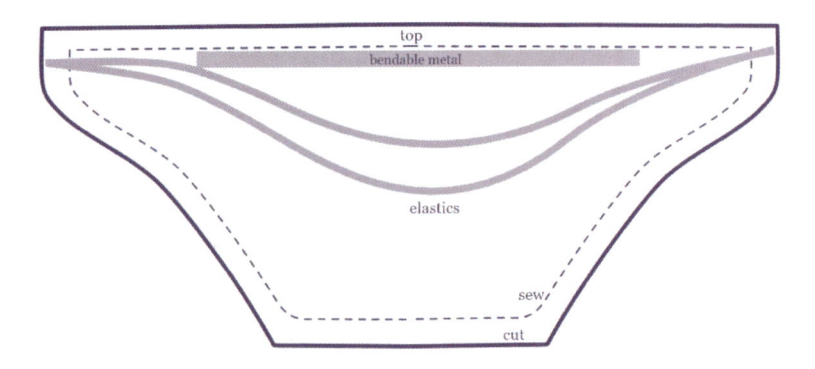

make sure elastic is lined up to the side of mask but should be slightly below top of mask. I then sewed down one side, across the bottom, then up the other side. I Stitch edge of elastic to mask.

9. Sew sides and bottom together.

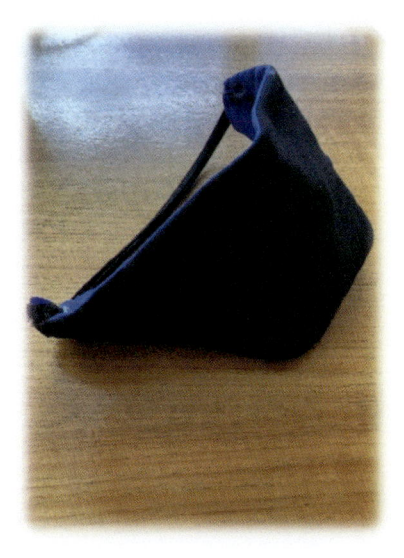

10. Mask is finished! Cut off any loose threads. Good job.

11. Can clean by steaming in instant pot steam/sterilization setting for 30 minutes.

Homemade Facemask Pattern

Regular sized mask pattern

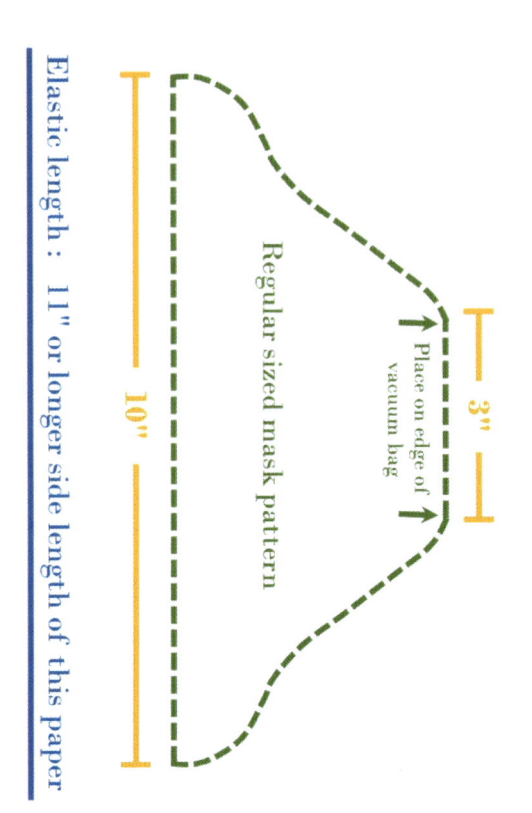

10"

3"

Place on edge of vacuum bag

Elastic length : 11" or longer side length of this paper

51

Elastic length : 10 1/2 "

8 1/2 "

Small sized mask pattern

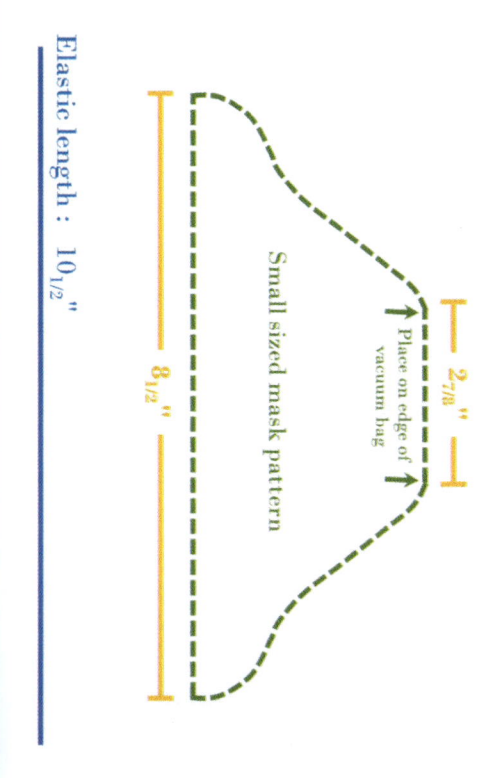

Place on edge of vacuum bag

2 7/8 "

Here is a link to download it

https://www.dropbox.com/s/dsj8lu9zi4uk3fk/mask%20patterns.pdf?dl=0

Some Tips: When You Can Not Find Suitable Materials for The Mask

If you do not find MERV 16 or HEPA filter, the best material for handmade masks is a double layer 100% cotton fabric that is tightly woven. Things like bedding and knit shirts are also decent options. If you donate masks, it is recommended that you avoid knit fabrics (e.g. T-Shirts) because they create holes when the virus is stretched through.

Be sure that products with hot water are prewashed to destroy sprouts and to pre-reduce material, so that it does not change shape until health workers themselves are washed.

I have talked to many healthcare professionals and it is clear that there are currently no precise guidelines or rules for the production of home-made masks for donations. Nevertheless, you should follow some best practices.

For the top of a sewing machine and cloth, you will need a nonwoven device that will help remove debris and metal (such as a paper clip) from the nose.

If you have good clothing or bedding at home, you can use it rather than buy new material.

NOTE: It was very difficult at this point to find elastic, so I marked * with the patterns underneath that use straps instead of elastic. Most designs use biased strap tape. You can buy bias tape, but it is actually very easy to make your own of the same fabric you use to make the mask (and this is better because it is 100% cotton).

Technically, cloth handmade masks are not hospital-approved, and some hospitals do not allow direct donations. Check with local hospitals in your area to see if they can use handmade masks

Bear in mind: not just hospitals require facial masks. Other facilities such as nursing homes and urgent care centers also tackle mask shortages when dealing with COVID-19 patients. Only non-health care staffs, such as veterinarians and firefighters, have no face masks and said that they support home-made models.

Other Suggestions: Facemask Patterns

Before handling your clean materials or sewing, make sure to wash your hands.

Recall testing and verifying if the company you are sewing needs a certain pattern. If

* Belt Pattern Mask

It uses belts instead of elastic, has a pocket to attach a filter and contains (optional) nasal wire. This seems like a Really GOOD model choice.

This face mask model was developed by the Turban Project and was shared by Deaconess Health Systems in their call for people to make masks.

This mask is incredibly simple to make – it starts with a tissue rectangle that is folded to resemble a surgical mask with elastic circling the face. If you have a sewing background, you can probably do each in about 15 minutes.

* Sweet Red Pappy Bias Tape Mask

This pattern is a great alternative because it uses biased tape straps, rather than elastic, which have become difficult to find.

This pattern is a great option. It is the same general design as the Deaconess mask but also contains a pocket that can be inserted by the healthcare provider. This mask is very similar to the deaconess mask and is also pretty straightforward to create.

* Fu Face Mask

This is yet another simple mask design – I have sewn up a couple of these now and will soon add a photo. This one has no plates, but is angled to provide good face coverage. The Fu Face Mask uses bias tape or tape for binding, so if you find it difficult to find elastic it is a good choice.

* A.B. Face mask

This facial mask was designed and shared by Jessica Nandino. It has plates in the front and links on the top of the head and on the bottom of the back.

This pattern takes a little more time to construct due to the connection of the ties, but also to the strong, comfortable fit. AND it has been designed to fit over a N95 mask and probably prolong their life.

This mask pattern is available in 4 sizes and uses elastic hair ties to go over the ears. The mask pattern is made in 4 sizes. It uses a contoured fit over the nose instead of platelets.

CONCLUSION

Homemade facial masks are highly recommended for the prevention of coronavirus. Home-made facial masks and face coatings are now approved to wear in public, from the hand-sewn tissues to bandanas and rubber bands.

Late last week, the Centers for Disease Control and Prevention released a revised guide to the public's wearing of facial covers, including home-made fabric masks. The updated statement comes as cases in the US and new data about COVID-19 transmission are published.

For months, the CDC has advised people suspected or confirmed ill with the COVID-19 to use medical-grade facial masks as well as emergency care staff. But spiking cases in the United States and especially in hotspots such as New York and Now New Jersey have shown that current policies are not powerful enough to flatten the curve.

There is also new evidence that a home-made mask can be used in crowded areas such as the supermarket, against no face cover at all. Significant attention is also paid to social distancing and hand washing.

The use of the masks by all people can provide some barrier protection against respiratory droplets coughed or sneezed around. Early reports indicate that the virus can spend up to one to three hours in the air after an infected person leaves the area. Covering the skin helps to keep these droplets from reaching and infecting others.

According to the American Lung Association, one in every four people diagnosed with COVID-19 may show mild or zero symptoms at all.

When you are around others, using a cloth face mask will help trap large particles that could be expelled through a tingling, sneezing, or accidentally began saliva (e.g. by speaking), which may delay transmission to others if you are not sure you are sick.

The American Lung Association says in a blog post that addresses the wearing of homemade masks, 'these masks are not intended to shield the wearer, but to defend it against accidental transmission – in case you are an Asymptomatic Carrier of Coronavirus.

The most important thing about the CDC message is that it is a 'voluntary public health measure' to cover your face on your way home and should not replace proven precautions, such as self-quarantine at home, social distances and hand washing thoroughly.

I hope and pray that manufacturers will be able to manufacture the medical grade face masks that are required by our health professionals! Meanwhile, making home-made facial masks as a last resort is one little thing that I can do to help during this tough time.

Printed in Great Britain
by Amazon